Introduction

This is the first in the **MyBones** series of condition-specific books for non-physicians, authored by board-certified orthopaedic surgeons. Each book focuses on a specific area: neck, back, hip, knee, shoulder, elbow, hand, ankle and foot along with several other topics that could be helpful to you. Please search on Amazon from time to time to see if a **MyBones** book addressing your area of concern has become available.

Medical science is complicated. When doctors talk, we use language uncommon to most people, even those highly educated in other disciplines. Thinking people wish to understand their medical problems. We hope that this booklet will provide you and your loved ones a better understanding of your diagnosis and options for treatment.

Two seasoned orthopaedic surgeons combine over 100 years of training and experience to help demystify the language of their profession. Moreover, they offer opinions on how they would wish their loved ones and themselves to be treated.

We believe this information will help you better communicate with your physician as well as enable you to ask relevant questions to get useful answers. We want you to avoid problems when possible and take an active role in helping your surgeon determine the best course to follow when help is needed.

Our training after university consisted of four years of medical school followed by five years of specialized training in orthopaedic surgery under intense supervision. After two years in the U.S. Navy, one went into academic surgery where he practiced orthopaedic surgery and trained future surgeons. After two years as an orthopaedic surgeon in the U.S. Air Force, the other joined a group of orthopaedic surgeons in private practice.

We take responsibility for what we say, but please remember that we are expressing our opinions based on training and experience. Medical science changes rapidly, so what seems to be true today may not appear to be so tomorrow. Furthermore, it is common for medical people to have different opinions, so your surgeon may have opinions different from ours. We are telling you what we think and believe to be true.

Reading this booklet does not make one an expert in the field. It cannot take the place of professional, in-person consultation. If your condition is persistent or worsening or you need more specific information about your case, please see an orthopaedic surgeon as soon as possible.

Be enlightened! Be empowered! Be healthy!

Table of Contents and Overview

Chapter 1: Causes of Hip Pain
Arthritis and tendonitis are common causes of hip pain; cancer and infection are much less common but highly consequential. Imaging studies (X-Rays, bone scans, CT scans, and MRI) are valuable in evaluating disorders and making treatment recommendations. Pain from the spine and poor circulation are cited.

Chapter 2: Non-Surgical Treatment of Hip Pain
Medications, injections, physical therapy and the benefits of walking aids are discussed.

Chapter 3: Surgical Treatment of Hip Pain
Total joint replacement is the most likely procedure for advanced arthritis and necrosis of the hip. Other procedures are briefly discussed, but total hip replacement is the likely choice. Chronic tendonitis may be due to a tendon tear that can be repaired. Chronic "bursitis" may actually be an undiagnosed tendon tear.

Chapter 4: Injuries of the Hip and Pelvis
Fractures of the hip are mostly fractures of the upper end of the femur. In most cases these require surgical treatment. The type of surgery generally depends on where the bone is fractured, but also the condition of the patient. Fractures of the pelvis in the elderly are usually associated with osteoporosis and rarely require surgery.

Glossary
Medical terms and phrases are defined to help our readers better understand the problems and treatments described.

Acknowledgements
We appreciate those who have inspired and helped us.

About the Authors
Brief biographers of the authors

Reviewer Comments
Commentaries by readers

Chapter 1
Common Causes of Hip Pain

Betty felt pain in her groin almost constantly. When she tried to walk, she had a marked limp and required a walker. She could not reach her feet to dress, and the lack of ability to maneuver her leg made personal hygiene difficult.

Hip Joint

Our weight-bearing joints degrade over time. Then they creak, squeak and ache, often to the point of becoming crippling. Fortunately, there are numerous ways to help make them better. Unfortunately, none is perfect.

The hip joint is a system of bones, cartilage, ligaments and muscles. The ends of the bones are covered with "articular cartilage", also known as "hyaline cartilage". The articular

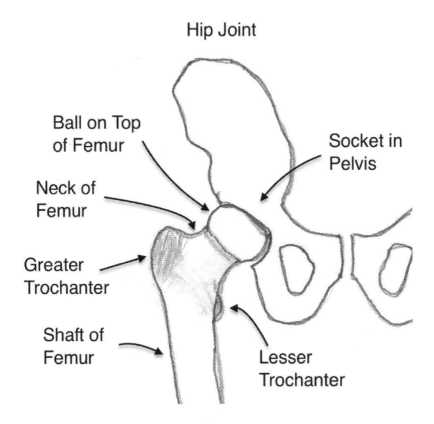

Hip Joint

Ball on Top of Femur

Socket in Pelvis

Neck of Femur

Greater Trochanter

Shaft of Femur

Lesser Trochanter

surface is a thin, firm, rubbery substance that provides a smooth, slippery surface. When "oiled" by fluid produced by the lining of the joint, the synovium, the surfaces of a joint touching each other are said to be more slippery than ice on ice. Age and "miles" cause those surfaces to wear. Injury, arthritis, and deformity cause them to wear faster.

Arthritis

In seniors, "wear-and-tear" arthritis, medically called "degenerative arthritis", is the most common cause of hip problems. Like most everything in the bone and joint system, there is a spectrum of wear from minimal to severe. In this discussion we are focusing on degenerative arthritis, whether it be from age, injury, or deformity.

Patients experience weakness, difficulty arising from a chair, trouble walking up and down steps, limited excursion of the hip and giving way that can lead to falls.

Limited range of hip joint movement is insidious in onset. If you have become unable to reach your toes for nail care or reach your foot to tie your shoes, it could be the result of stiffness in the hip due to arthritis. Inability to cross one's legs or to lie flat in the facedown position is common.

Normal Hip Joint as Seen on X-Ray

Arthritic Hip Joint as Seen on X-ray

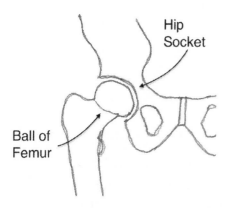
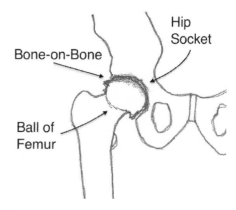

Hip Socket

Ball of Femur

Bone-on-Bone

Hip Socket

Ball of Femur

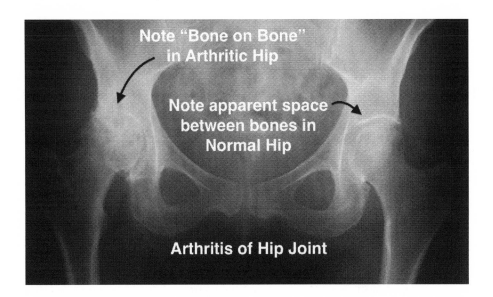

Note "Bone on Bone" in Arthritic Hip

Note apparent space between bones in Normal Hip

Arthritis of Hip Joint

True hip joint pain typically occurs in the front of the thigh or groin, but it can be felt in the buttocks or side of the hip as well. The pain is often felt down the front of the thigh toward the knee, and patients often think they have a knee problem when they are actually experiencing hip pain referred to the knee. Sometimes hip and thigh pain originates in the back and is due to irritated spinal nerves.

Necrosis of the Femoral Head
Sam had been a heavy drinker for many years. One day he noticed aching in his groin. It was not too bad at first and after a few months seemed to be getting better. Suddenly, it markedly worsened. His pain was tolerable at rest, but walking made him miserable. Not only did he feel pain, but he could also feel grinding in his groin area when standing up or walking. X-rays showed flattening of the femoral head due to collapse of the upper aspect of the ball.

Loss of the blood supply to the femoral head goes by a variety of names: "aseptic necrosis", meaning it is not due to infection; "avascular necrosis", meaning it is due to loss of blood supply to the ball; and "osteonecrosis", simply meaning bone has died. Fractures of the femoral neck and dislocations of the hip, which are discussed in Chapter 4, can cause necrosis of the femoral head. Regular, heavy alcohol intake is associated with necrosis as is regular use of the cortisone category of medications. When we do not know the cause, we call it "idiopathic". No matter the cause, when the femoral head collapses, the joint surfaces no longer fit smoothly together and painful arthritis ensues.

Osteonecrosis of the Femoral Head

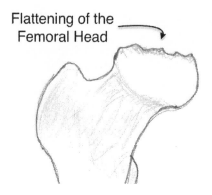

Flattening of the Femoral Head

Tendonitis and Bursitis of the Hip
They rolled John into my clinic in a wheel chair. Seventy-plus years old, he had suffered hip pain since he leapt from a Jeep as a twenty-year-old soldier. He had managed to complete his twenty years to retirement in the U.S. Army, but his pain had relentlessly worsened. Despite multiple, non-surgical treatments, his increasing symptoms required a walking cane, then crutches and finally a wheel chair.

Upon examination, his pain and tenderness were not in the groin but on the side of the "hip" over the greater trochanter, the bony prominence that one can feel on the side of the hip. He had excellent range of motion of his hip and no groin pain with any direction that we maneuvered it. He had no back pain or indication that the pain was referred from elsewhere. His x-rays showed minimal arthritis, not nearly enough to account for his pain. John was desperate to walk again and was disappointed when we told him that a "hip joint replacement" would not fix his problem. After carefully considering more non-surgical

8

treatments, which had previously not worked, we operated. We were surprised to find a large tear in the tendon of the gluteus medius muscle where it attaches to the greater trochanter. This large, powerful muscle is essential to stabilizing the hip when walking. We repaired it. With time and physical therapy, he resumed walking with only a cane for assistance and was pleased with the outcome.

His MRI had originally been reported as normal. A radiologist highly skilled in bone, joint, and muscle imaging disagreed. He saw signs of muscle loss that we later found to be consistent with tears of the gluteus medius and minimus tendons in multiple other patients.

Description of Hip Joint and Muscles: The femur is the bone that extends from the hip joint to the knee joint. At the top is the ball that fits into a socket in the pelvis comprising the hip joint. The side of the hip that we can feel with our fingers is the greater trochanter. The hip joint is buried deep in tissues and not detectable by touch. The gluteus medius and minimus muscles that move the limbs apart, such as in spreading one's legs, keep our bodies from sagging when walking. They arise from the pelvis and attach to the top and the sides of the greater trochanter. With tendonitis, frequently associated with a tear of the gluteus medius and minimus tendons, there will be tenderness on the side of the hip along with pain and weakness with walking.

X-rays may be normal or show some degree of arthritis. MRI does not always show the tear itself, but in chronic cases MRI typically reveals muscle loss in the gluteus medius and minimus muscles as secondary evidence of such a tear.

Hip Tendon Tears

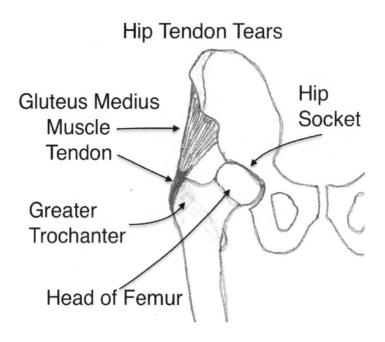

Gluteus Medius Muscle

Hip Socket

Tendon

Greater Trochanter

Head of Femur

Bursitis: Patients with "trochanteric bursitis" typically have pain when pressure is applied to the side of the hip such as when lying on their side. They may limp. The examiner would find tenderness over the greater trochanteric bursa. Visible redness or swelling over this bursa may or may not be visible.

X-rays may show a normal appearing hip joint but there could be some evidence of arthritis, as well. If arthritis is seen on an x-ray, the pain may be disproportionate to the amount of arthritis. MRI is done when the symptoms are unusually severe or chronic. In bursitis, one would see fluid in the bursa, but not the extensive muscle loss seen with a tendon tear. Some combination of arthritis, tendonitis, and bursitis can coexist.

In the unusual case where, along with pain, there is redness and swelling over the greater trochanter, infection should be considered. When this occurs, we typically aspirate fluid, extract it through a needle, for analysis.

Trochanteric Bursitis

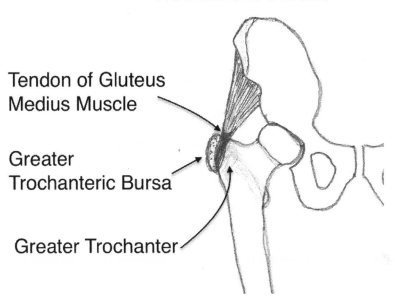

Tendon of Gluteus
Medius Muscle

Greater
Trochanteric Bursa

Greater Trochanter

Cancer

Primary bone cancer, cancer originating in bone, is unusual in seniors. More likely it would be metastatic from cancer that spread to the bone from elsewhere. Initially, there may be no symptoms, but in advanced cases the pain could be severe and constant. A distinguishing characteristic is that pain from an arthritic hip may subside when sitting or lying down but bone cancer pain would likely continue. One of our regular questions to patients was about the presence of night pain. Did it awaken them for no apparent reason? This is not specific for cancer, but one should be aware of it as a possibility. Hip pain from arthritis can awaken people, too, but that probably has more to do with position or movement than the deep aching pain people experience with cancer.

In the early stages there are often no physical findings such as limitation of motion, tenderness, swelling, and redness.

A high index of suspicion, especially if the patient has or has been treated for cancer, aids in diagnosis. X-rays are helpful in finding areas of bone that appear to be more or less dense than normal. Fortunately we have mirror image sides of our skeletons, so we can always compare one side to the other. Unfortunately, there must be about 25% loss of bone mineral for a defect to appear on x-ray, so other studies are often needed in the early stages.

Cancer can weaken bone to the point of fracture. If someone with known cancer, such as breast or lung, suffers a broken bone without a fall or other obvious reason, cancer should be high on the list of possible reasons.

An excellent test for bone cancer is a bone scan where the radiologist injects a radioactive dye into the blood stream and then does a scan of the entire skeleton to see if there are areas that show up as "hot spots", sites where the radioactivity is concentrated. Do not worry about the radiation. It is less than what one would get from having a chest x-ray. CT scans are helpful in detecting bone defects but are not as good as MRI in imaging marrow and soft tissue changes.

Blood tests, such as a white blood cell count to evaluate for leukemia and other blood studies that reflect increased bone activity, are useful.

Infection
Sarah, a middle aged woman who had taken cortisone medicines for years for COPD, chronic obstructive pulmonary disease, was admitted to the hospital with pneumonia. With aggressive antibiotic and pulmonary therapy, her pneumonia got better but she continued to worsen overall. She could not move her hip without severe pain. She had tenderness in the groin. X-rays appeared normal except for the vague appearance of some swelling about the hip. MRI had not been invented.

Hip joint infection is unusual in adults unless there has been a severe injury exposing broken bone to the outside or from a surgical wound infection, especially in the presence of "foreign material" such as artificial joints or devices used to stabilize fractures. In people with compromised immune systems, such as those with HIV or those on chronic cortisone therapy, the chance of infection is increased. Typically this infection would come through the blood stream from an infected organ such as a lung with pneumonia or other infection elsewhere. Tuberculosis, TB, is now uncommon except in those with compromised immune symptoms. TB does not typically cause the redness, heat, and pain associated with bacterial infections.

Symptoms of infection are pain, fever, and swelling. Blood tests are usually consistent with infection. The same array of studies noted for cancer (x-rays, bone scan, CT scan, MRI) is also helpful in diagnosing infection. Ultimately your physician needs to know exactly which organism is causing the infection, so a sample is needed. If there is fluid in a joint or an abscess from which fluid can be drawn with a needle that should suffice. If not, then a biopsy of the involved bone is indicated.

A word of caution: If you think you have a bone or joint infection, do <u>not</u> start yourself on a random antibiotic that you have cloistered in your bathroom cabinet. Taking antibiotics before a sample has been collected can disrupt the laboratory results even though that particular antibiotic may not be effective in fighting that infection. Thus, your physician would have to guess which antibiotic to use or hold off a few days and then take another sample while the infection continues to inflict damage unimpeded.

Referred Pain from the Spine
Back pain is commonly "referred" to the buttocks. As the buttocks are commonly called the "hip", patients often say that they have hip pain when it is actually pain originating in the back.

This can be confusing because pinched-nerve pain can also be felt in the buttocks, the groin, and the front of the thigh. Physicians can usually determine the source of pain by taking a history and performing a physical examination, but not always. Also, spine and hip joint problems can co-exist, making distinguishing one source from the other difficult.

Vascular Pain

We must also consider a blood vessel origin for buttocks pain. If the arteries are clogged, one can have buttocks pain, especially with walking or other exercise. Part of the physical examination should include evaluating the circulation in the extremities.

Chapter 2
Non-Surgical Treatment of Arthritis, Tendonitis, & Bursitis

Non-Surgical Treatment of Hip Arthritis

Oral Medications
Over-the-counter (OTC) medications such as the non-steroidal-anti-inflammatory medications (NSAIDs) such as ibuprofen and naproxen, or acetaminophen are usually sufficient. These medications, however, are not without potentially serious side effects and can unfavorably interact with other medications, especially anticoagulants, "blood thinners". Check with your physician or pharmacist before taking them.

The cortisone category of drugs can make you feel much better but the side effects can be serious, especially when taken in high doses or for long periods of time. Those side effects can include bleeding in your stomach and intestines and possible long-term damage to the hip and shoulder joints.

We know of no side effect from taking glucosamine/chondroitin sulfate, so physicians do not generally object to your taking it. Some people get great relief and others get none. We suggest trying it for three to six months and then deciding to continue based on whether you think it is helping.

Injections
Occasional injections of cortisone type medications make sense if the pain is intermittently intolerable and for major events such as trips or family occasions where you really need to walk. They are also useful if you have medical problems so severe that surgery is not an option. The risk of serious side effects, however, requires us to be careful about doing this too often.

Exercises

Strengthening exercises for the hip can improve your gait and ability to stand. One should work on the abductors, the muscles that move the limb out to the side, and the extensors, those that move the limb backward.

Stretching is important. Many older people walk with very short steps. Some of this could be poor balance and fear of falling, but some is also likely due to hip stiffness. Be sure to work on spreading your legs and on bending your hip by bringing your knee to your chest. Extension, straightening the hip, is difficult but lying face down on a firm surface will help. Pushing the thigh backward helps to straighten the hip as opposed to letting it stay in a bent position all of the time.

Bicycling and swimming are excellent ways to retain hip mobility, may reduce pain and are generally good conditioning exercises.

Walking aids

Seniors do not like to appear old. Using a cane is a giveaway. Using a cane or a stick in the hand on the <u>side opposite the bad hip</u>, however, can work wonders. The reason this works is a little complicated, so just give it a try and see for yourself. Shifting weight to the cane can lessen pain and smooth one's gait. It seems counterintuitive, but for the same reason you may be able to walk better by carrying heavier items like suitcases or groceries on the <u>same side as the bad hip</u>.

A walker is more stable than a cane and can be used to reduce pressure on the hip joint. The deciding factor for using a walker, of course, is to allow ambulation while avoiding falling.

If the pain is not too severe and a cane is not needed, adding a half-inch shoe lift on the good side can take a little weight off the bad hip and may make it less painful.

Non-Surgical Treatment of Hip Tendonitis and Bursitis

Initially, the treatment for these two conditions is the same. The idea is to relieve pain; self-treatment with heat or ice may be all that you need. The decision to use ice or heat is difficult to make in advance. We recommend trying both and then using whichever works. Be alert to avoid heat burns and cold injury to your skin. The skin should be protected from ice with a few layers of towels and by limiting the ice application to twenty minutes or less per session. You can do this frequently, but do not reapply ice until the feeling in the skin has returned.

If that is insufficient, a physical therapist can apply ultrasound to the area. Ultrasound creates heat by "exciting" molecules in the deeper tissues. If you have metal in the area, such as a hip pin or prosthesis, you should not use ultrasound.

Over the counter medications such as the anti-inflammatory medications and acetaminophen can be effective. Because of the potential for serious side effects, we do not recommend oral cortisone type medications for tendonitis or bursitis of the hip.

Cortisone injection is a common and helpful treatment and can seemingly "fix" the problem. All injections carry the risk of infection; furthermore, cortisone injections have weakening effects on tendons. Thus, too many injections could have a negative effect. We recommend limiting such injections to no more often than every three months. If two or three do not resolve the issue, then further evaluation is needed.

Bursitis could be due to a bacterial infection. If the area is red and hot, a needle should be inserted to remove fluid for testing. If an infection is found, it may be satisfactorily treated with antibiotics alone, but if that does not work, then it may require incision and drainage.

Takeaways

1. Arthritis, tendonitis, and bursitis can be treated non-surgically.
2. The symptoms of bursitis and tendonitis can be successfully treated for long periods of time without surgery.
3. Arthritis with damage to the cartilage cover of the joint surfaces will not be cured, but the symptoms can be reduced to a tolerable level for long periods of time without surgery.
4. Arthritis symptoms naturally wax and wane, so treatment may not be the only reason for improvement.
5. If tendonitis or bursitis does not subside with the above treatments, one should consider further evaluation for a tendon tear or infected bursa.

Chapter 3
Surgical Treatment

Deciding whether to have elective hip surgery for arthritis and tendonitis

No matter how bad your pain, arthritis and tendonitis do not threaten your life. It is reasonable to tolerate the symptoms rather than have major surgery. Because only you can determine the severity of your pain and impairment, only you can make that decision.

When discussing surgery, we explained to our patients what to expect in the short and long terms and the potential consequences. When decision time came, we asked for a definitive answer from the patient. "Yes", meant yes, proceed with surgery. "No", meant no, and "maybe" also meant no. For those who were not sure they were ready to proceed, we advised them to wait until they were unequivocally ready.

It is rarely "too late" to get better, so there is generally no reason to "rush" into elective surgery.

Hip Joint Surgery

What the surgeon should decide

Your surgeon is better prepared to determine what surgery is best, the type of prosthesis to use, and the type of incision to make. If you do not trust your surgeon, you should seek another. This is not to discourage you from asking questions of your surgeon. You should learn all you can and be comfortable with the surgeon's reasoning and recommendations before agreeing to have surgery.

What the patient should decide

In deciding whether to have surgery, you may wish to consider the following:

Pain: The pain is unbearable and keeps you from sleeping, walking even short distances, or going to work.

Quality of life: You cannot perform reasonable activities such as playing golf and walking for exercise. Running and jumping are not options after hip joint replacement; do not use those as reasons to have joint replacement.

Surgery: We strongly encourage you to first pursue non-surgical treatments. They can really help, so you should give them a chance. There may come a time, however, when non-surgical treatments are insufficient, and you want to do more. Although joint replacement is overwhelmingly the most preferred option in older people, we want you to be aware of the other treatments outlined below:

Arthroscopic Surgery: This entails inserting a small diameter metal tube onto which a video camera is mounted and surgical instruments through small incisions into the joint. Modern technology has made visualization of the hip good, and different types of surgery can be accomplished. Removing debris from wear and tear and trimming of the labrum, a structure similar to the "cartilage" of the knee, are the usual reasons. In a condition called "impingement", bone can be trimmed away from the rim of the socket. Removing "bone spurs", however, is unlikely to be helpful since that does not address the basic problem.

Osteotomy: The femur below the ball can be cut and reoriented so that a less arthritic part of the ball presents itself to the hip socket. Before replacement was so well developed, this was frequently done. Osteotomy would be uncommon these days, especially in older people, since joint replacement typically works quite well.

Girdlestone Procedure: In certain cases, such as an otherwise incurable infection when all other treatments have failed, the ball and neck of the femur can be removed. The patient is left with a partly functional extremity, but poor control of the hip requires a walker or crutches.

Arthrodesis: Surgeons can initiate the process to make the two bones of the hip joint to grow together. This was often performed before joint replacement had been refined. The inconvenience of being unable to move the hip makes this undesirable. It is still an option, however, when joint replacement is inappropriate, such as in the face of incurable infection.

"Joint Replacement": Although commonly called joint replacement, it only involves replacing the surfaces of the bones. You still need your muscles and ligaments to make it work. That said; the joint replacement procedure is usually life changing by reducing pain and allowing one to return to more normal activities.

Decompression and bone grafting for osteonecrosis: In the early stages, before collapse of the top of the femoral head has occurred, osteonecrosis can be treated by such techniques as drilling holes into the femoral head and by insertion of a vascularized bone graft. These procedures are generally done to preserve the natural hip in younger people. In older people, however, we recommend total hip replacement.

Incision and Drainage: Joint infections typically require more than just taking antibiotics. The pus needs to be removed. The classic method is I & D, incision and drainage, that entails making an incision to drain the fluid and thoroughly irrigating the joint. Dead tissues are removed. This can be done arthroscopically as well. A drain, rubber or plastic tube, is placed into the joint and out through the skin to keep excess fluid from collecting. Once the drainage subsides, the drain can be removed.

Types of devices (prostheses) used in "hip joint replacement"

Partial Hip Replacement: If the socket is in good shape, only the ball is replaced and the patient's own socket is used. This is most often done for fractures in patients too feeble to undergo "total" joint replacement and who are expected to have low ambulatory demands.

Total Hip Replacement: The ball on top of the femur is replaced and an artificial cup is inserted into the damaged socket.

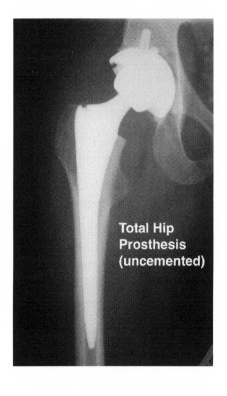

Total Hip Prosthesis (uncemented)

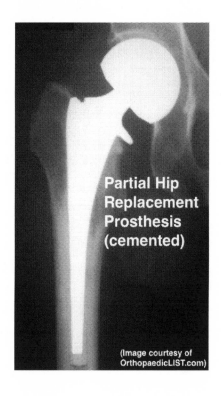

Partial Hip Replacement Prosthesis (cemented)

(Image courtesy of OrthopaedicLIST.com)

Is using cement preferable? Your surgeon will decide whether to use a special cement to secure one or both parts of the prosthesis. Cement works well but has a greater potential for loosening after several years. Non-cemented fixation is generally preferable, but if your bone is weak, driving a tightly fitted stem into the shaft of the femur could cause it to fracture.

Bearing surfaces: There is an ongoing discussion about the best types of artificial joint surfaces to be used. To date, the most reliable surfaces are a metal ball and a special plastic liner locked into a metal-backed cup. Ceramic and metal-on-metal components are not necessarily optimal.

How good can it be? If successful, you can regain excellent range of motion, and the ability to walk normally with little or no pain.

Can it make you worse? Unfortunately, yes, and you need to know what could happen. Fortunately, the chance of any of these problems is low, but the consequences are great. We take them seriously. The potential for the following complications keeps surgeons awake at night:

Infection: No matter how hard the surgical team tries, we cannot prevent infections every time. Treatment for an infected hip replacement involves aggressive antibiotic therapy and additional surgery. Often the prosthesis has to be removed, while the infection in being eradicated, followed by an additional surgery to insert a new one.

Metal allergy: Most people with metal allergies are allergic to nickel. The high quality metals used in joint replacement are very low in nickel and allergies to them are uncommon. "Rejection" of a prosthesis due to metal allergy is unusual. If a prosthesis were to be "rejected", an indolent infection should also be considered.

DVT (deep vein thrombosis), also known as "blood clots in the legs": DVT causes pain and swelling in the legs. Such a clot can break away from the vein wall and migrate into the heart to be pumped into the lungs (pulmonary embolus). This can cause serious breathing problems, even death.

Nerve injury: As they surround the hip joint, three nerves are of particular interest (sciatic nerve, femoral nerve, and pudendal nerve). Any could be damaged during hip replacement.

Persistent pain after hip replacement
Despite everything going well during and after surgery, some people keep on hurting, and some develop pain months or years later. Here are some, but not all, potential causes:

Loose prosthesis: Most prostheses used today have special surfaces designed to allow bone to grow into those surfaces, like vine on a trellis. On rare occasions bony ingrowth fails to occur, resulting in groin or thigh pain from micro-motion between the prosthesis and the bone. Diagnosis is difficult but x-rays and MRI can be helpful. As a last resort, surgical exploration can be considered. Late loosening is more likely to occur with prostheses that were cemented into place. Although this creates a tight and secure fit, bone can resorb away from the cement over time, also resulting in painful loosening. Micro-motion is difficult to see on imaging studies but, if the stem of the prosthesis becomes grossly loose, one can sometimes see a conclusive, "windshield-wiper" effect. If the prosthesis is loose, it will need to be replaced.

Infection: Aggressive bacteria can cause obvious infection that becomes apparent soon after surgery. Others, however, can be much less aggressive and cause indolent infections that are not obvious. If there was even a suspicion of infection in the early post operative period, such as drainage that was greater than expected or what may have been called a "superficial infection" that subsided with antibiotics, and there is persistent pain after surgery, deep infection should be considered. Loosening, as noted above, may be caused by infection. Treatment of deep infection generally involves removing the prosthesis and adjacent damaged tissues to the extent possible and replacing the prosthesis. Our preference would be to initially replace the prosthesis with temporary components, try to ablate the infection with antibiotics, and insert a new prosthesis once the infection has been cured. Some excellent surgeons, however, advocate inserting the final prosthesis during what is called a one-stage procedure and then trying to cure the infection with antibiotics.

Tendonitis: In an unpublished study of 100 total hip replacements, we found that 25% of patients had some degree of undiagnosed tearing of their gluteus medius tendons. This condition is discussed later in this book. Tears can also occur after surgery. If one has persistent pain on the side of the hip after total hip replacement, tendonitis should be considered.

Referred pain: If the pain is in the buttocks area, it may be referred from the spine and not related to hip replacement surgery.

What can you do to help yourself in advance of surgery?
Check with your primary care physician to be sure you do not have anything that needs to be evaluated or corrected before surgery. Do not wait until the last minute.

Build strength in your muscles, especially your hip abductors and extensors.

Infection prevention
    Have all dental work (cavities, gum disease, broken or loose teeth, and cleaning) definitively treated well in advance. Bacteria from dental diseases or procedures can

enter the blood stream and cause infection around your new joint. Ask your dentist to determine the possible need for antibiotics during your surgery and subsequent dental work.

Be sure your facility checks for potentially serious bacteria in your system. A nasal swab can be used to check for MRSA, methicillin resistant staphylococcus aureus, which can cause joint infections. Other sources of infection such as urinary tract infection should be discovered and cured well in advance of surgery. Make sure you do not have infections or sores in your skin. If so, get these resolved before proceeding.

Shower the night before and the morning of surgery.

Prepare your living facilities for when you return home. For example, remove trip hazards such as throw rugs. Secure loose electrical cords and toilet seat extensions.

Some things to expect after surgery

The leading concerns in the immediate period after surgery are pneumonia, DVT, and infection:

Lying in bed on strong pain medications predisposes us to pulmonary congestion that could lead to pneumonia. Thus, you will be asked to sit up, walk frequently, and use a breathing device to help inflate your lungs.

Multiple efforts to prevent DVT are begun. Mechanical prevention with intermittently inflating sleeves on the legs to propel blood flow toward the trunk, compression stockings, and elevation of the legs are implemented. Anticoagulants, commonly known as "blood thinners", are used to help prevent excessive clotting. You will be asked to help by working your ankles up and down to push blood from your veins toward your heart, to walk frequently, and to elevate your legs.

Despite diligent sterilization of instruments and prostheses; using preparations to kill bacteria on the skin to be incised; isolating the operative area with sterile drapes; operative team hand scrubbing; use of gowns, gloves, caps, masks, face shields, and "space suites"; managing operating room air exchanges; and administering antibiotics just before surgery, wound infections still occur. Fortunately, the infection rate is below 2%, so your chance of infection is low. Should infection occur, you would need prolonged antibiotics and surgical procedures to help eradicate it.

Other concerns include bleeding, other hospital acquired infections, urinary retention and constipation. Bleeding is typically well controlled, but if you bleed too much, you will need a blood transfusion. Urinary catheters can allow bacteria into the bladder resulting in urinary tract infections. They are typically used during surgery and then removed soon thereafter. Not only is a urinary tract infection serious, but also if infection gets into the blood stream from the bladder or elsewhere, it can settle around the prosthesis and cause a wound infection.

In older men, with enlargement of the prostate gland, urinary retention is common. Lying in bed and taking pain medications makes this worse. Getting up to void and reducing the intake of pain medicine can help. Recatheterization may be required.

Constipation is not considered a complication but a result of inactivity and pain medications. Stool softeners are generally started right after surgery, but as long as you are taking opioids the likelihood of constipation is high.

Potential Complications with the Hip Prosthesis

Until the body has a chance to rebuild the tough fibrous capsule around the new hip, there is a possibility that the ball will dislocate; that is, slip out of the socket. Your surgeon will let you know if there is a risk of this happening and what you should do to prevent it.

Leg length differences are common concerns. Sometimes the surgeon must use a longer prosthesis to make the hip tight enough to stay in the socket. This may result in a slightly longer leg. If so, a shoe lift on the opposite side will compensate for it. Sometimes patients misperceive that the new hip has been made longer than it should be, but that could be because it was functioning as shorter before the surgery. If the leg has been shortened due to degeneration of the hip joint with loss of height from narrowing of the joint space, deformity of the head of the femur, or contractures preventing the hip from fully straightening before the surgery, it may seem longer than it actually is following replacement. Once the body adjusts to the limb returning to normal length and the patient regains adequate muscle strength to stabilize the pelvis with weight bearing, this sensation typically subsides. Finally, keep in mind that a one-half-inch difference in leg lengths is normal for adult humans.

With modern metallurgy, total hip prostheses are very unlikely to break. On the other hand, ceramic components were thought to be a great way to reduce friction and wear. They worked great in laboratories and clinical trials. Then a few malfunctioned. Many years ago, the ceramic femoral head component in one of our patients shattered. The pieces had to be removed surgically and replaced with a metal ball. He did well, but having repeat surgery is no picnic, and the risks of complications are ever present. We have never seen such an issue with metal prostheses and the uncommon breakage problem with ceramic prostheses seems to have been solved.

What can you do to help yourself immediately after surgery?
Pay attention to what your surgeon tells you to do and do it.

Use gravity to help reduce swelling in your legs. Edema is mostly water, and water runs downhill. Avoid prolonged standing or sitting with your operative leg hanging down. When not walking, sit or lie down with your foot higher than your knee and your knee higher than your hip.

Tighten your calf and thigh muscles frequently, and work your feet up and down at the ankles. This "calf pump" mechanism can help keep blood flowing to prevent DVT.

What can you do to help yourself after you have recovered from surgery?
Avoid running and jumping as well as sudden starts and stops. These activities can cause loosening of the prosthesis-joint interface and prematurely wear the plastic portion of the joint, like wearing the brake pads in your car.

Maintain good oral hygiene, focusing on your teeth and gums. Medications can cause dry mouth with a lack of saliva. Use an over-the-counter, sugar-free saliva substitute to help prevent decay and gum disease.

Notify your primary care physician if you have signs of infection anywhere in your body, and get it treated promptly. There is urgency in preventing bacteria from spreading through your blood stream to your artificial joint.

Do not put yourself at risk. Avoid falls, especially from heights. Stay off ladders and countertops. Wear stable and secure shoes that are easy to put on. Use walking aids such as a cane, walking stick, or walker if necessary. Fractures around artificial joints are very challenging and can permanently diminish the functionality of your new joint.

Work at regaining a normal gait. Strengthen your hip muscles. Watch yourself walk in a mirror or store window and ask friends and family to tell you when you limp. Using a cane until you can walk without limping can help you relearn a normal gait rather than being left with a chronic limp.

Be patient. People are not machines. A joint replacement is not like getting a new tire for your automobile and immediately speeding down the interstate highway. You can walk, but it will not be immediately normal. Rapid recovery is highly touted, but we always told our patients that it took six weeks to start feeling good, six months to really begin enjoying their new joints, and at least a year to reach maximum improvement. This is not to discourage but to reassure you that if you have not completely recovered in three weeks or three months, there is still plenty of time to improve.

Surgical Treatment of Tendonitis and Bursitis of the Hip

Bursitis of the hip rarely requires surgical treatment. If it is infected, incision and drainage may be necessary. Sometimes those with conditions like rheumatoid arthritis may need to have the bursa removed. Otherwise, non-surgical treatment should suffice.

Tendonitis is likely a tear in the gluteus medius tendon attachment to the greater trochanter, a condition that causes chronic hip pain. If conservative treatments have not worked and severe symptoms have persisted for six months or more, MRI is recommended. If there is atrophy in the gluteal muscles with or without a visible tendon tear, then surgery should be considered. The torn tendon should be reattached to the bone and given eight weeks to heal before one resumes weight bearing. Afterwards, patients should use a cane or crutch in the hand opposite the affected hip until they are able to walk without pain or limp. Muscle strengthening is essential, but regaining strength takes extra time due to longstanding muscle weakness.

Surgical Treatment of Infection of the Hip Joint

Incision and drainage have been discussed above. In the case of Sarah, the lady with a hip infection that was most likely a complication of her pneumonia, we performed incision and drainage. Despite improvement in her lungs, she was worsening overall, so something needed to be done. After a few days the drainage diminished and became clear, so the drain was removed. She survived, but her hip joint became arthritic due to the infection. She wisely decided to accept the arthritis over a total hip replacement. Having already had an infection in that joint and her propensity for infection dramatically increased her chances of having another infection in her hip, this time with the additional burden of a foreign body, her artificial hip, in the infected area. Foreign bodies in infected tissues make curing them extremely difficult.

Caveats

Obesity: Excessive body weight makes surgery and recovery more difficult, and obese patients are more likely to have complications and less satisfactory results. It behooves patients to get into the best physical shape possible before surgery and continue that program afterwards.

Referred pain: Hip joint pain is often "referred" to the knee. Sometimes patients are adamant that the problem is in their knees rather than their hips despite clinical evidence that the hip is the greater problem. Sometimes x-rays show that both the hip and the knee are arthritic. In that case, we recommend that the hip replacement be done first. Often, replacing the hip will resolve both the hip and knee pain. In contrast, replacing the knee is unlikely to resolve hip pain.

Takeaways

1. Hip surgery, except for fractures and infection, is elective. You do not have to have it. If you are not sure you are ready, that means you are not ready.
2. Hip joint pain is typically felt in the groin, but can include the buttocks or side of the hip. Buttocks pain without groin pain is likely referred from the spine. Side-of-hip pain without groin pain is usually due to tendonitis or bursitis.
3. Your role is to decide whether you are ready to have surgery, but your surgeon is the most knowledgeable about what to do, what type of prosthesis to use, and the best methods to perform the procedure.
4. Complications from hip replacement surgery are serious but, since the incidence of serious complications is low, your chances of doing well are high.
5. It takes months to recover from major surgery, so do not despair if you have not recovered as much as you wish until at least a year after surgery.
6. An artificial joint is not a natural joint. You need to make concessions and take care of your artificial joint to make it last.
7. Tears of the tendons attaching to the greater trochanter have only been recognized in the past few years. Their existence is not well known, even among orthopaedic surgeons. Persistent pain on the side of the hip and not in the groin, especially in view of relatively normal x-rays, needs to be evaluated with MRI. Severe arthritis and tendon tears at the greater trochanter can co-exist.

Chapter 4
Injuries

Opal was headed to the kitchen when she slipped on a throw rug and fell. She was in severe pain and could not get up. She lay on the floor until the next morning when her daughter called, and she did not answer. Fortunately her daughter lived in the same city and was able to check on her. She was not OK. Her daughter called 911, and Opal was taken to the hospital. Soon thereafter she had surgery to replace the ball of her hip joint.

Royce, a healthy, athletic man in his forties, was an avid biker. He struck a curb at high speed and was thrown off. Upon recovering his senses he found himself lying on the ground in excruciating pain. He was taken to the hospital where he had surgical stabilization of his fracture.

Anatomy of the Upper Femur

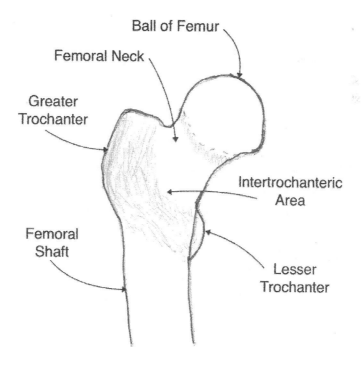

What is the difference? Opal simply slipped and fell. She should not have suffered a hip fracture. Royce, on the other hand, suffered significant trauma. Anyone crashing a bicycle at thirty miles per hour would be expected to have a serious injury.

Both had fractures of their upper femurs. Their balls and sockets were undamaged, so theirs were not "hip joint" fractures. Their fractures were near but did not directly involve their hip joints. Nevertheless, common terminology categorized them as hip fractures.

Types of Fractures

It is possible to suffer fractures of the hip socket, but they are rare and likely to occur from events like high impact motor vehicle crashes. Fractures of the head, "ball", of the femur are also very uncommon and generally associated with hip dislocations. The typical fractures affecting seniors are

1. Fractures of the femoral neck: fractures between the ball and the trochanters,
2. Intertrochanteric fractures: fractures through the upper part of the femur between and often including the greater and lesser trochanters, and
3. Fractures of the pelvis.

Fractures of the femoral neck

For most fractures of the femoral neck, the usual recommendation is to replace the ball with an artificial one so the patient can immediately bear weight. Inserting pins or screws across the fracture can be done, but there is inadequate bone on the ball side for strong fixation, thus requiring the patient to be either non-weight-bearing or partial-weight-bearing until the fracture heals. This is not practical for older people. The high-energy requirement to ambulate with crutches and walkers limits what they can do and increases the chances of disrupting the fracture by their accidently putting too much weight on that leg. Also, the blood supply to the femoral head is tenuous, so even if the fracture heals, the head of the femur may have lost its nourishment resulting in dead bone that would crumble over time. That would require a second operation to remove the pins and perform a replacement.

The pressing question is whether to perform a replacement of only the ball or to replace both the ball and socket, total hip replacement. For low activity people, replacing the ball is generally satisfactory. If the person is healthy and vigorous, then a total hip replacement is more likely to provide a better outcome, even though it takes more surgery.

Opal had a femoral neck fracture. She was not very active. Her bone was osteoporotic. Internal fixation was not appropriate. The ball was replaced. She was up with a walker the next day and able to return to her previous status in a few weeks.

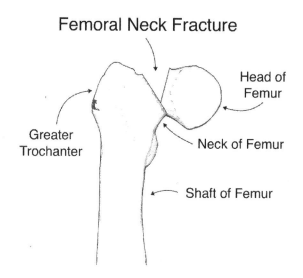

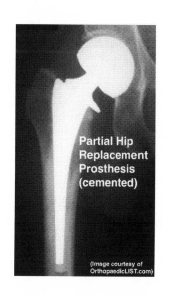

As shown in the above x-ray example, the ball has been replaced, but you may wonder why there is such a long stem going into the femur. Think about a trailer hitch on a car. A lot of force is applied to the ball by the trailer, so a strong supporting mechanism is needed to keep it from breaking off. The same goes for the ball of the femur.

Fractures in the upper femur below the femoral neck

Intertrochanteric Fractures: Fractures in the area of the trochanters, are typically treated with a large screw inserted through the femoral neck into the femoral head. The screw is then attached to the shaft with a rod inside the femur or a plate screwed to the side of the femoral shaft.

Royce, the biker, had an intertrochanteric fracture. This was internally fixed with a plate and screws, and he was out of bed on crutches the next morning. Within a couple of months his fractures had healed and he resumed biking, albeit with more care and less gusto. Discomfort caused by rubbing of muscle and tendon on the side of the plate was resolved a year after injury by removing the plate and screws. The bone had united, so he did not need the internal fixation device any longer.

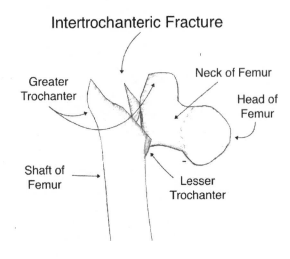

Intertrochanteric Fracture

Greater Trochanter

Neck of Femur

Head of Femur

Shaft of Femur

Lesser Trochanter

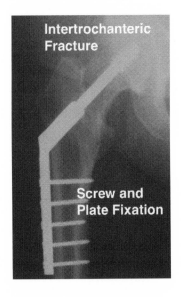

Intertrochanteric Fracture

Screw and Plate Fixation

Base of Neck and Subtrochanteric Fractures: These occur at the very bottom of the femoral neck and just below the lesser trochanter in the upper few inches of the shaft of the femur. Both are often slow to heal and place enormous stress on the fixation devices for a long time. Treatment is typically a rod inserted into the shaft of the femur with a screw or screws running through the rod and then through the femoral neck into the head of the femur.

Subtrochanteric Fracture

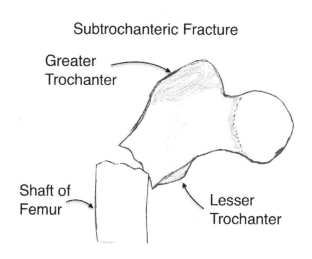

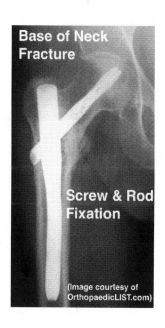

"Internal fixation", stabilizing the fractured bone with a device implanted into the body, is intended to reduce pain and allow the patient to start moving. Procedures to do this began in the 1940s when studies showed a high mortality rate for patients who had to lie in bed for months until their fractures healed. Furthermore, these fractures were followed by a high rate of incapacitation since the bones did not heal in the proper position. Now, we stabilize bones to positions as normal as possible so that patients can get out of bed and begin walking to help avoid bedsores, pneumonia, and DVT, and have functional limbs afterwards. Internal fixation devices act as internal casts to hold the bones in place until they heal. Replacements with artificial balls and sockets are also used to reduce pain and mobilize patients, but as these prostheses become integral parts of the joint, fracture healing is not required. The condition of the patient and the location of the fracture determine what device to use.

Fractures of the pelvis

Great Aunt Bessie lived alone in a small town far removed from medical centers. She fell at home and lay on her sofa for six weeks until her grandniece brought her to see us in a wheel chair. X-rays showed a couple of healed fractures in her pelvic bones. When we told her it was again safe to resume walking, she sashayed out of our clinic pushing her own wheel chair.

Older people with fragile bones can break their pelvis with simple falls. Usually the bones remain in adequate position and require no treatment other than reduction of weight bearing until the fractures unite. Bessie was fortunate that she did not have a potentially disabling fracture of the "hip", and her self-treatment worked just fine.

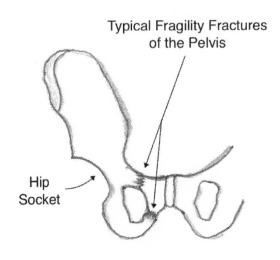

Typical Fragility Fractures
of the Pelvis

Hip
Socket

Dislocations

Dislocations of the hip in older people are uncommon, partly because our bones are the weaker link and tend to break before soft tissues tear allowing the ball to be forced out of the joint.

A dislocation is most likely to occur in a motor vehicle crash in which an occupant's knee strikes the dashboard with the hip bent about ninety degrees. If the bones do not break first, the ball can be pushed out the back of the socket. Surgeons put the ball back into the socket, typically requiring general or spinal anesthesia. That is usually sufficient, but sometimes the ball crumbles many months later from damage to the blood supply, or arthritis results from damage to the articular surfaces of the ball and socket.

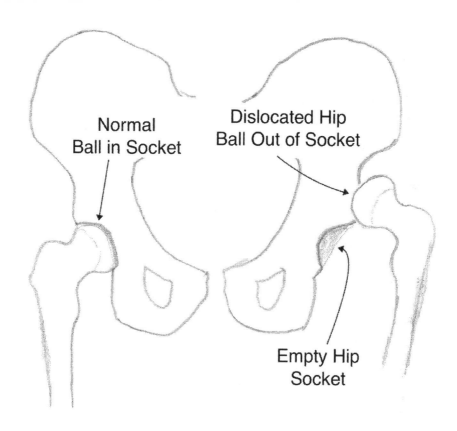

Normal
Ball in Socket

Dislocated Hip
Ball Out of Socket

Empty Hip
Socket

Takeaways

1. "Hip fractures" are actually breaks of the upper parts of the femur, the bone that runs from the hip to the knee.
2. Surgical treatment is almost always done to reduce pain, restore function, and to mobilize the patient to help avoid complications such as pneumonia, DVT, and bedsores.
3. The type of surgery depends on what part of the bone has been fractured and the condition of the patient.
4. Fractures of the pelvis in seniors are typically fragility fractures from osteoporosis in those with falls that would not otherwise cause fractures. Surgery is rarely required.
5. Prevention and treatment of osteoporosis, avoiding risky behavior, and "fall proofing" one's home can help people avoid fractures.

Glossary

Positions of Body Parts

Proximal and Distal: Relates to the location of one body part toward or away from another body part

    Proximal: Closer to the trunk or body part in discussion

        Example: In the lower extremity, the knee is proximal to the ankle.

    Distal: Further from the trunk or body part in discussion

        Example: In the lower extremity, the ankle is distal to the knee.

Superior and Inferior: Above and below. By convention, the person is considered to be in the "The Anatomic Position" (i.e. vertical with arms down by the sides).

    Superior: Above

        Example: The head is superior to the chest.

    Inferior: Below

        Example: The neck is inferior to the head.

Medial and Lateral: Relates to the sagittal plane of the body (the plane that "divides" the body into right and left portions)

    Medial: Toward the middle of the body (the sagittal plane) relative to some other body part

        Example: The naval is medial to the side of the body.

    Lateral: Away from the middle of the body (the sagittal plane)

        Example: The side of the body is lateral to the naval.

Anterior and Posterior: Relates to the coronal plane of the body (the plane that "divides" the body into the front (ventral) and back (dorsal) portions

    Anterior: Toward the front of the body relative to another part or parts

        Example: The toes are anterior to the heel.

Posterior: Toward the back of the body relative to another part or parts

    Example: The heel is posterior to the toes.

Flexion and Extension

Flexion: The bend of an extremity or the spine at a joint or joints

    Degrees of Flexion: The "neutral position" of the knee (and other joints) is considered straight. When one is sitting in a chair with the feet on the floor the knees are in approximately 90° of flexion.

    Dorsiflexion and Plantar flexion: When the foot is pointed downward, the ankle is in "plantar flexion". When the foot in pointed upward (such as when the heel is on the floor and the forefoot is lifted) it is in "dorsiflexion".

Extension: The opposite of flexion of an extremity or spine at a joint or joints.

    Hyperextension: Passing beyond the neutral position and going into an overextended position

        Examples

        When the knee is "bent backwards", it is hyperextended.

        When the wrist is bent backwards, it is hyperextended.

        When one leans backward beyond the usual erect position of the spine, the spine is in hyperextension.

Tendons, Ligaments, and Bursae

Tendon and Muscle: The continuation of a muscle that attaches the muscle to bone

Muscles are attached to bone in at least two places, and these attachments are through a transition of the beefy muscle tissues into tendons. Tendons can be long and cable-like or so short that the beefy part of the muscle appears to be attached to bone. The tendon attachment to bone is an actual blending of the tendon tissue into the tendinous tissue within bone (collagen) that is analogous to steel mesh in concrete. They attach above and below a joint so that when they contract, they move the joint. Muscles move joints by actively shortening (contracting). To allow a joint to move, they relax on the side opposite the side on which the muscles contract. That is all they can do. Muscles contract on the flexion side of a joint to bend it, and contract on the extension side to straighten it.

Ligament: Very similar in structure to tendons, but ligaments are the tough structures that hold bones together to make joints. Like tendons, ligaments can be long and round like cables or short and wide and a variety of shapes in between.

Bursa: Envision a plastic bag that is moistened with a thin layer of oil inside. Then move the surfaces of the bag back and forth over each other to sense the low resistance. Bursae are similar. They are pouches with smooth inner surfaces and contain oil provided by the body. They are found in areas where tendons and ligaments rub back and forth over bone, reducing friction at those spots. When normal, they are flattened and assume the shape of the structures around them. When abnormal, they swell with fluid and become painful.

Injuries

Fracture: Broken bone
> **Comminuted fracture:** The bone is broken into more than two pieces. It could be three pieces or 3,000 pieces but if it is more than two it is comminuted.
> **Simple fracture:** Not comminuted, or skin is not broken, or both of the above

Compound fracture / Open fracture: The skin is torn open.

Angulated fracture: The bone fragments are bent in relation to each other.

Displaced fracture: The bones at the fracture site are offset in relation to each other. It is common for displaced fractures to also be angulated.

Greenstick fracture: Fractures in children whose bones are "softer" than those of adults and bend without breaking apart. This is due to a higher percentage of collagen vs. calcium crystal in children than in adults. They are likened to immature tree limbs ("green sticks") that bend but do not snap in two as would dry, brittle ones.

Fragility fractures: A fractures that occurs in those with fragile bones such as those of people with osteoporosis. These are typically fractures of the "hip" and "wrist" and "compression fractures" of the spine. Adults who suffer any of these fractures should be tested for osteoporosis.

Fracture Patterns

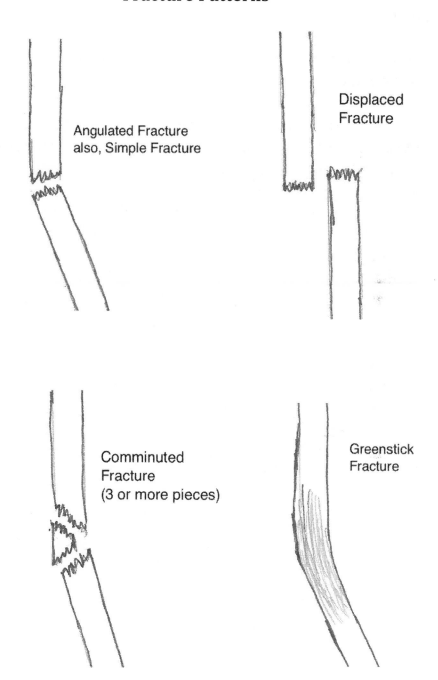

Angulated Fracture
also, Simple Fracture

Displaced
Fracture

Comminuted
Fracture
(3 or more pieces)

Greenstick
Fracture

Dislocation and Subluxation

Dislocation: The disruption of a joint such that no part of a joint surface remains in contact with the opposite joint surface

The often-used phrase "complete dislocation" is redundant since the term dislocation means that it is complete.

Fracture-dislocation: A situation where the bones comprising the joint are broken as part of the overall injury resulting in dislocation

Thus, there is a fracture and a dislocation in the structures that comprise the joint.

Subluxation: A partial disruption of a joint where some parts of the opposing joint surfaces remain in contact

> **Example**: When a shoulder "partially goes out" it is subluxed.

Imaging Studies

MRI (Magnetic Resonance Imaging): An image generated by a machine that uses powerful electromagnets to intermittently cause atoms in the body to misalign and then realign resulting in an emission of electromagnetic rays. MRI demonstrates both bone and soft tissues and helps define abnormalities.

CT Scan (CAT Scan, computerized axial tomography): Special computerized x-ray machines that provide much greater detail of bone and soft tissues than regular x-rays

Bone Scan: Imaging test that uses radioactive dye injected into the subject's vein. A special dye is taken up preferentially by bone. If the bone is more active than normal, more dye will be taken up and a "hot spot" will appear on the image. The whole body is typically scanned making this a good study to use when looking for bone cancer. Increased dye uptake is also seen during and long after fracture healing.

Diagnostic Ultrasound: Ultrasound can be used to produce images by bouncing sound waves off of soft tissues and bones. These studies require expert operators and can be performed quickly. The images are not as distinct as those of MRI.

DVT Prevention

Anticoagulation

The phrase "blood thinning" is commonly used, but it is misleading. It suggests that you have diluted the blood, which would make the patient anemic without accomplishing the intent. In order to reduce undesirable clotting (coagulation) of blood, we use "anticoagulants" that interfere with clotting mechanisms. To prevent DVT, deep vein thrombosis, after surgery, physicians partially anticoagulate their patients' blood for a few weeks. In some cases, patients need to be "fully anticoagulated", which puts them at greater risk of excessive bleeding from the surgical area and from minor injuries or lacerations.

Calf Pump

The heart pumps blood downhill under high pressure. Blood then passes through a bed of capillaries before having to flow uphill to return to the heart. Imagine pumping a liquid downhill where it must flow through a sponge before returning to the pump several feet higher than the sponge. Also called the "second heart", the "calf pump" is an elegant mechanism. The veins below the knees have soft walls and run among the muscles of the calf. When those muscles tighten, they squeeze the veins forcing the blood to flow away. At the thigh level those same veins have valves that direct the blood upward toward the heart. A result of malfunctioning valves is "varicose veins" that occur when the valves fail to keep blood from flowing backward (downhill) causing increased venous pressure. The veins dilate, become visible, and the legs swell.

Acknowledgements

We cannot possibly thank enough everyone who helped and inspired us along the way. Our wives have steadfastly stood beside us and in our places many times for many years. We thank them from the bottom of our hearts. Without them, our careers as well as our lives outside of work would have been meaningless.

We owe a profound thanks to those who helped educate us: Our teachers in grammar school, high school, university, and medical school, and the professors in our orthopaedic training programs, all of whom gave so much of themselves to help us learn and understand our profession.

Special thanks go to novelist and acclaimed Professor of Orthopaedic Surgery Laurence Dahners, M.D. for his recommendations and assistance in publishing this book.

We deeply appreciate our volunteer readers who worked diligently to help make this book more readable and understandable: Linda Hundley, Sandra Elam, Marie Gillis, Kenneth Dickinson, and Jack Kuske. Any errors you find are ours, but without our readers there would be many more.

Finally, we greatly appreciate your reading this work. As it is the first in a series, we would like to hear from you about what you like and do not like, so we can try to improve with each book. Posting a review on Amazon would be most appreciated.

Many thanks!

About the Authors

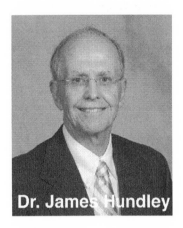

James D. Hundley, M.D. is a graduate of the University of the North Carolina School of Medicine and the Orthopaedic Surgery Residency Program of UNC Hospitals. After completing his orthopaedic training, he served as an orthopaedic surgeon in the U.S. Air Force for two years before joining an orthopaedic group practice in Wilmington, N.C.

His primary medical interests were in sports medicine where he was a university athletic team physician for over twenty years and adult reconstruction (primarily hip and knee replacement surgery). Retired from medical practice, he continues to operate OrthopaedicLIST.com, a resource for orthopaedic surgeons founded in 2003.

Hundley's peers in orthopaedic surgery, the UNC School of Medicine, UNC-Wilmington, his community, and his state have recognized him for his efforts. He continues to serve on non-profit boards and a foundation focused on community health.

His writings include multiple scientific papers published in medical journals, numerous magazine articles, and two blogs: www.agingdocs.com and http://www.orthopaediclist.com/blog.

Hundley and his wife, to whom he has been happily married for fifty years, have three children and five beautiful granddaughters. His other interests include golf, fishing, and reading.

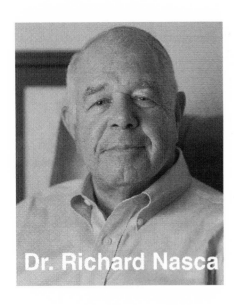
Dr. Richard Nasca

Richard J. Nasca, M.D. was born in Elmira NY and is a graduate of Georgetown College and Georgetown Medical School. He completed his internship at the Hospital of the University of Pennsylvania and postgraduate training in Surgery and Orthopaedics at Duke University and Affiliated Hospitals.

Dr. Nasca served as Chief of the Amputee and Hand Services at the Philadelphia Naval Hospital caring for Vietnam casualties.

Dr. Nasca held teaching appointments in Orthopaedic Surgery at the University of Arkansas School of Medicine and the University of Alabama School of Medicine. During his time in practice he specialized in caring for patients with spine deformities, injuries and disorders.

He has been married to Carol T. Smith, R.N. for fifty-two years and has three children and one granddaughter. Dr. Nasca lives in Wilmington N.C. He is a volunteer physician at local medical clinics, on Advisory Boards at the College of Health and Human Services at University of North Carolina at Wilmington and has published five books, several book chapters and seventy peer reviewed scientific articles.

Dr. Nasca works in the soup kitchen and does fund raising for the Good Shepherd Center, is involved with the First Tee program as a coach, and is a certified Master Gardener. He enjoys golf, gardening, swimming and travelling.

Reviewer Comments

"The information in this book is for inquisitive people seeking compact, direct, understandable, and unambiguous information relating to hip problems. The authors are vastly experienced, thus affording them the ability to provide a very practical discussion on the subject. It should be required reading for those with hip issues."

----Kenneth D.

"What a wonderful resource for laymen like me! I have been puzzled by my pain, which started in my groin, for two years now! I thought I had pulled a muscle or it was a disc in my back.......... The pictures are very helpful and I have a much better understanding of why I thought it was my back that was failing......... The section on whether to have surgery or not is again, very clear and helpful......... So, I am glad to be able to justify why I am not ready for surgery. And I also have a much better idea of when it will be time to have the surgery."...........

----Martha B.

"Hip pain so bad that you finally go to the doctor, but you don't understand what the doctor is telling you about your condition. This booklet will not only clear that up, but it will help you to know what questions to ask."

----Jack K.

"Often patients see doctors and then try to explain to family and friends the information given them. Many times the information becomes garbled. This book will help both patients and support groups to have access to reliable information explained in layman terms. I highly recommend."

----Sandra E.

Made in United States
Orlando, FL
23 December 2022

27619874R00033